HEALTH, YOUTH
AND BEAUTY
THROUGH
COLOR BREATHING

Books by Linda Clark

HEALTH, YOUTH AND BEAUTY THROUGH COLOR BREATHING

LINDA CLARK

YVONNE MARTINE

Celestial Arts
Berkeley, California

NOTICE:

Neither the author nor the publisher make any claims, direct or implied, for any of the procedures mentioned in this book. No allegations as to the therapeutic properties of any of these procedures are made or intended.

The reader should consult a duly licensed physician for any condition that logically requires his services.

Copyright © 1976 by Linda Clark and Yvonne Martine

Celestial Arts
P.O. Box 7327
Berkeley, California 94707

First Printing, February 1976
Made in the United States of America

Library of Congress Cataloging in Publication Data

Clark, Linda A
  Health, youth, and beauty through color breathing.

  Includes index.
  1. Breathing exercises. 2. Color-Psychology.
3. Hygiene. 4. Beauty, Personal. I. Martine,
Yvonne, 1923– joint author. II. Title.
RA782.C56 613.1'92 75-28754
ISBN 0-89087-113-2 pbk.

    9 10 11 – 87

CONTENTS

Like beauty, color is in the eye of the beholder. For that reason, the colors shown on the back cover of this book can only approximate the shade and intensity of individual desire and effectiveness.

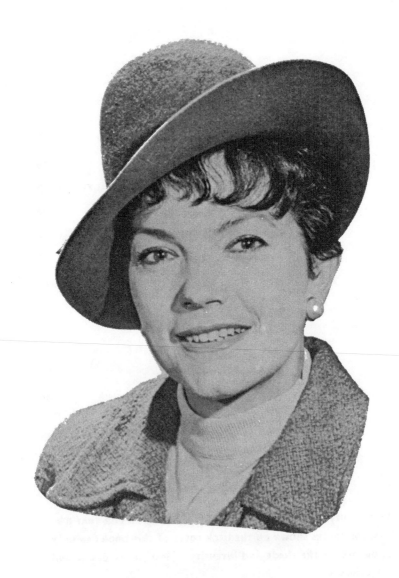

YVONNE 1961

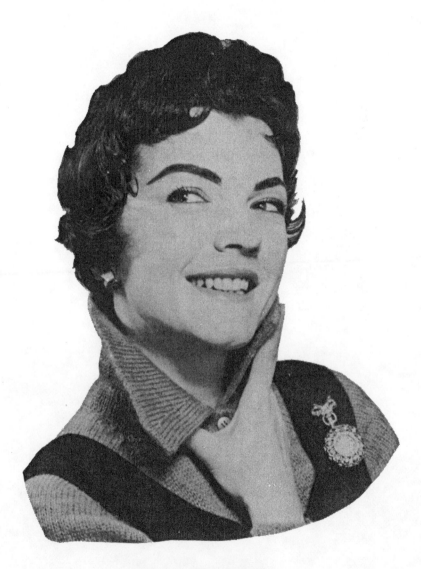

Yvonne Today

1.

iNTRoduciNG
yVONNE

Scarcely a year has passed since I (Linda Clark) and my co-author (Yvonne Martine) first met. The circumstances of our meeting and how this book came to be written are quite unusual.

For years I have researched, compiled information and written books and articles concerning natural methods of achieving and maintaining health, youth and beauty, frequently exploring color.

While writing my book, *Color Therapy*,[1] I was greatly frustrated because the medical monopoly seems to be fighting any method of healing which does not coincide with their "consensus of opinion." This does not necessarily mean that the type of healing under consideration is dangerous, useless or wrong; but because it does not meet with their consensus or agreement, they refuse to accept it or to allow it to be practiced, perhaps because they fear its competition. At any rate, I was warned that I must not include any method of using color for healing, which involved equipment of any kind in the book, no matter how successful, because the medical monopoly had already outlawed not only such equipment but the practitioners who used it. Since I am always trying to find help for suffering humanity, such edicts are hard to take. But I had no choice: I could *not* include the information!

And then a strange thing happened.

I was actually at the post office, ready to mail the finished manuscript to the publisher, and I picked up the incoming mail first. A heavy envelope addressed to me caught my eye. It had been sent by someone whom I did not know nor had ever heard of. I opened it and saw with a gasp, an article about how it is possible to help yourself by *breathing* color. I read the article, a photocopy from a magazine, and realized that here was a last minute reprieve. The medical monopoly might be able to stop us from using color healing equipment, but it couldn't stop us from breathing! So I hurriedly included the article with the manuscript and shipped both off to the publisher.

That article had been written by Keith Ayling, about

Yvonne Martine, who had discovered the effects of rejuve nation by breathing and thinking color. As a model herself, and the head of a modeling school, she had proved in her own case, as well as with her students, that it could be done. I will explain later how she does it, and how she learned the technique. Meanwhile, with permission of the author, the article was incorporated into my book in a chapter entitled, "Thinking Pink." It explains briefly the method as well as how to get more results from this technique. Some people had tried and failed. Other people lost interest and gave it up altogether. But those who persevered obtained results of various kinds. One woman said she lost nine pounds by this method without changing her diet one iota. But others asked, "Isn't there more information, not included in that chapter, to help us achieve more definite results?"

There *is* more information to help your success with this method, and that is why this book has been written. Everyone wants to get rid of wrinkles, bags under their eyes, feel better and look more youthful as each ages in years (which need not include aging in appearance). So I got in touch with Yvonne, who lives in Indiana, and asked her if she could help. She consented and the following informa- tion is the result. Prior to this, when I published the original chapter about her, I talked with people who had met her and I requested before-and-after pictures to assure me the whole thing wasn't just a hoax. But before beginning this book, she flew from Indiana to California to see me and I found that she is indeed the proof of her own pudding. Although she is well over fifty, she looks about thirty, with nary a wrinkle or eye bag or a pound of excess weight. She is real! Before giving you the method she had used and still uses, I want to introduce her as a person, so you will understand what makes her "tick" and why she says some of the things she does to explain her method.

Yvonne is a mystic in the sense that she is, and always has been interested in the "unseen," including the occult, the esoteric, metaphysics, as well as the Bible, together with the benign influences of the saints, masters, angels,[2] and other helpers. She is spiritually oriented, but not spiritualistic. All of her life she has studied and read every word she can get her hands on to throw light on all of these subjects. For some reason, she says, she has also always been interested in color, its vibrations, and the resulting effect upon our lives. This sum-total of knowledge she has acquired is not only quite impressive, but completely self-taught, and was the preface to her vision which started her "thinking pink" which was followed by such surprising results.

I will let her take up her own story from here, in her own words.

"I am not a healer, or a medium, or even a dietician," she says. "I am merely an ordinary woman who started out in the entertainment field as a singer, later became a model, a fashion newswriter, TV and radio broadcaster, and I now conduct a modeling school.

"My home life may surprise you when I admit that I have been widowed once and divorced twice, and am now happily remarried. I am not only a mother of three sons, at this writing aged nine, twenty-four and thirty, but I am a grandmother as well. I run my own house and continue with my career, which adds up to a busy but wonderfully satisfying life, largely because I feel that I am helping others.

"I am five feet, one inch tall, weigh ninety-eight pounds, and happy to report that I do not have a wrinkle on my face. My figure is probably better than it was when I was twenty-five."

I (Linda) can testify to this, since although over fifty, Yvonne really does not look over thirty, has a youthful face plus a well stacked figure, although, as you will see, this was not always so.

As long as she can remember, Yvonne has always had a horror of aging. As she watched her parents and friends age, she thought there must be some way out and she was determined to find it. She was sure there was a clue, and she kept searching for it. She dug into hundreds of books, journals and articles. She found that there were famous beauties who had maintained their youthful appearance until they died, but the reasons given included secret potions, exercises, even the effects of heredity. Yvonne was almost sure there was something more.

Meanwhile, she was nearing forty and aging was beginning to catch up with *her!* She was developing wrinkles, eye bags, a sagging chin and hated to look into a mirror. She watched other women with similar problems, who, in panic, were rushing from one beauty salon to another, or from one diet to another, all without much effect. She redoubled her search, but still did not find an answer.

About this time, her beloved first husband died, leaving her with two children to raise and support. She was looking and feeling worse as well as despondent over her loss and new responsibilities. But she still drove herself in search for the "fountain of youth and beauty." She read, she worried, she prayed.

Then, one day, without warning, it came. I will let Yvonne explain what happened.

"It was almost midnight one August night, and I was lying in bed, reading as usual. My house is surrounded with a thicket of trees; no house or street lights are visible. Suddenly I looked out the window to see, set against a velvety black background of night, a tiny pulsating pink dot. As I watched in amazement, it rounded out to about four or five inches in diameter, and was an indescribably beautiful shade of pink with just a hint of orchid. As I watched, it arched a little to the left of the window screen, and then flattened out a bit. I thought, it can't be a flying saucer; it's too small. And if it were, it would have become entangled in the trees.

"I was completely mystified. I asked friends, ministers, clairvoyants, even a medium. No luck. Nobody knew. Then I began to wonder if I had really seen it, or if my mind was playing tricks on me. I went to a psychiatrist. He didn't accept or reject my vision; he merely gave me a clean bill of mental health and a verdict of being *normal*.

"One day two months later, as I was doing the breakfast dishes, the explanation hit me like a flash. I *had it!* The message came loud and clear in my mind that *breathing that shade of pink would erase wrinkles*, as well as change my figure.

"Now that I had the clue, I didn't know what to do with it. But I meditated and asked for help and gradually it came. Directions for breathing pink were given to me bit by bit and the puzzle fell into place. I began to practice it with fervor, believe me! I will give you a step-by-step formula in the next chapter. While I was spending ten minutes daily practicing this new technique, friends began to stop me and exclaim over my changing appearance. They told me I looked *different*, or asked me if I had discovered a magic diet. They seemed puzzled and thought I was fibbing when I said I just felt extra well. I wasn't ready to share my information until I was sure I had all the answers. Actually, complete results did not come over night, but improvement was obvious along the way, and eventually my wrinkles and eye bags departed, and have not returned. My figure improved, too. The complete transformation took nine months in all, but it has been worth it. By this time my students were clamoring for similar help which I finally shared with them. The method has worked for others, too.

"This morning I opened a letter from one of my pupils which read:

I still cannot believe what has happened to me. Halfway through your lessons I began to change all over. As I told you when I first saw you, I had pills for everything. But one morning I awoke feeling glad to be alive for the first time in years. No kidding! I settled down to my morning color breathing and I caught sight of a woman in the mirror. It looked like me but it wasn't me any more, but a woman who reminded me of myself years back before the bags and wrinkles and worry lines took over. I didn't need any pills that morning. And I haven't taken any since. As for all those aches and pains I used to carry with me, not forgetting the

> extra pounds with which I was overloaded; they have gone too.
>
> And something else. It works, Yvonne, it works! My daughter says she is getting jealous of me, looking so young. And I'm in love again with my husband who left me six months ago because he couldn't stand me, anymore than I could stand myself.

Yvonne continues, "When this woman came to my class for the first time, she was a good thirty pounds overweight and plagued with assorted aches and pains. She was utterly miserable, hating herself and the entire world. But she changed the whole picture. I have a sheaf of similar letters from hundreds of friends and students who, by devoting a few minutes a day to correct color breathing, men as well as women, have made themselves over, which surprised them as well as their friends. Wrinkles and bags from faces, and rolls of fat from bodies have all responded to this method of breathing pink. It is done anytime, anywhere, even when driving or getting ready for bed.

"Here is another example: Mrs. B.L., one of my pupils, came to me originally, a plump, unhappy looking blonde who admitted she was approaching her thirty- fifth birthday, although she looked fifty-ish. She told me very frankly that she was bored with her husband and married life. She suspected that he didn't love her anymore, and said she didn't blame him.

> I'm just a fat old duck; even my husband thinks so. So if you have anything to help me, I'm willing to try.

Mrs. B.L. learned to breathe pink every single day

and later wrote me:

> It's wonderful. My husband loves me again and I love him, too. You have changed my whole life. I have even taken a job. I couldn't get one before because I looked too old and fat and my feet hurt. Now I enjoy every minute of the day.

"Let me show you how you can learn to breathe color correctly, too, first for youth and beauty, and later for health."

2.

why
color
works

Obviously, many people are going to pooh-pooh the idea of the effect of color on the human body. The information in *Color Therapy*, with reports by scientists, doctors and others who have studied color and done extensive research with it, will prove an eye opener to such scoffers. Not only that, those who have already tried the color breathing technique without visible results need to learn both the laws of color as well as how to apply them through breathing it *properly. Shortcuts will not work!* Nor will a *lick-and-a-promise* approach. You cannot learn to swim, play the piano or drive a car in a haphazard manner. You must work at it *consistently* in order to be successful. Here are certain facts and rules which also must be observed in learning color breathing in order to assure success.

Sound and electricity are invisible. Color is visible. Furthermore, each color and shade has its own specific wave length or frequency. When these wave lengths impinge upon the eye or the body, something happens. Dr. John Ott found that when light, which is a source of all colors, reaches the eyes, it does not stop there; it penetrates the body where it stimulates certain glands. This explains why chickens which are awakened early in the morning by exposure to light lay more eggs.

Dr. Ott has also learned, after years of research associated with his time-lapse photography for Walt Disney Studios, that different colors can produce different effects on flowers, plants and people. The findings are laboratory proved and *physiological*, not psychological, although psychological effects of color do exist.

So color is just another form of wave length. We should not sell any form of wave length short, since different forms produce telephone, radio, TV, radar, laser beam and a host of other miracles.

Our forefathers, who would never have believed that telephone, radio, TV, even automobiles and airplanes could be possible or a part of our daily life routine, would have scoffed in derision at such *nonsense*. Today we take such things for granted. It behooves us to maintain an open mind. Pooh-poohers often end up red-faced.

In addition to the fact that color has wave lengths which can affect living tissue, it is time to take a look at something else which has been around a long time, but which is beginning to attract attention for many newcomers. This is metaphysics. There are countless groups who have long studied metaphysics, whereas others are just getting around to it. Yoga is a prime example. Yoga students who meditated regularly, formerly were considered peculiar. Now, it seems, everyone is meditating. Classes of instruction are springing up everywhere, even on college campuses. But metaphysics is not limited to yoga; it is a part of many groups. Metaphysics is learning what the mind can do.

Metaphysical students are taught that mind can affect the body and that thoughts can become things. Metaphysical students are also taught that each person has more than one body, which is physical and visible. There are, apparently, other bodies, like interweaving envelopes, which surround or penetrate the physical body, but which only those privileged people with X-ray vision can see. There are several bodies, too technical to include in this discussion, except for one, which all metaphysical teachers agree is highly important for everyday living. This body is known as the etheric body.

The etheric body is an exact duplicate, metaphysicians say, of the physical body, but vibrates at a much higher, lighter rate than the grosser denser physical body. Some research has discovered that disease may often register in the etheric body before it actually appears in the physical since the physical body is a copy-cat and produces, eventually, whatever first appears in the etheric. The beautiful part of the etheric system is that *you can influence your own physical body, either for health or appearance, through the etheric body!* You can give it a blueprint to use, and since the physical body is considered the servant of the etheric, it will faithfully reproduce these blueprint conditions in your physical body once that blueprint pattern is complete, and accepted.

How do you influence the etheric body? *Mind is the builder.* Thoughts have vibrations—weak or strong, good or bad, depending upon you who control them, and if properly presented to the etheric, can, in turn, influence your etheric and physical bodies accordingly. You have already heard the statement,"Thoughts are things". Metaphysicians go even further. They maintain that you are the sum total of your thinking, dating back to hours or years ago, depending upon how you influenced your etheric body at some previous time. You may not accept this; for example, that you are sick today because of what you thought several weeks, months or years ago. But a thought might well have crept in when you weren't looking, especially if it were accompanied by a strong feeling such as fear, which not only impresses the etheric body deeply, but also galvanizes the subconscious mind into action, a powerful combination in shaping your future.

For example, often (though not always due to extenuating circumstances) health specialists die of their own speciality. One world renowned heart specialist recently died of a heart attack. Cancer specialists have died of cancer. The reason: they think about these subjects constantly, which impresses their etheric body and if accompanied by fear , is relayed first to the subconscious, the part of the mind which reacts to feeling of any kind, thence to the physical body. One man, whose parents died within a few weeks of each other of cancer, stated ominously, "I will also die of cancer in ten years." He did! This is why the Christian Scientists have a word for it which, according to their belief, reads, "Put porter at the door of thoughts." They don't believe in taking chances. And neither should we.

We know a woman who refuses to speak a negative word, or think a negative thought. She learned this rule the hard way after discovering that whatever she said or thought eventually set up a pattern of cause and effect, and she did not like the effects. When she started thinking positively only, her life definitely improved.

So now we are beginning to get a glimpse of how we, ourselves, can get results with our own etheric and physical bodies.

We must visualize what we want; NOT what we don't want! Visualization gets our desired blueprint across to the etheric body. We must repeat this again and again until the blueprint has taken hold in the etheric so the idea will later be picked up by the physical body. Since thought has vibration, we must *think* what we want, as well as *visualize* it *strongly*. Wishy-washy thinking never accomplishes anything but wishy-washy results. And since color is also vibratory and can affect living tissue, we can add color to thought for further success. This is like thinking in technicolor.

This approach gives us an exciting concept to use. But we must be cautious that we do not fall into certain traps which delay our progress.

Scientists tell us that the physical body is constantly trying to renew itself, given a chance. We are learning that we *must* include proper nutrition as well as proper thinking. Also, the blueprint you construct for your etheric body to influence your physical body *must* be a positive blueprint (including what you want, only) as well as be used positively. If you change the blueprint to a negative one which includes the way you look now, or worse yet, the way you *don't* want to look, one day, and oscillate back and forth, back and forth, between that and your new bright and shining blueprint of what you wish to accomplish, like programming a computer, you are going to jam the works and get nothing at all. Confusion is going to set in and your programming etheric body computer is just going to give up, and you can't blame it.

You also need to program your blueprint regularly, as well as consistently. Do it daily until results begin to show, indicating that the message has gotten through and can begin to change your body cells according to your specifications.

Yvonne reports that although she noticed improvement soon after she began her own program, it took eight more months before the program was completed with final, perfect results. She says she has known others who took three years for results, depending upon their application, regularity and consistency, as well as their ability to concentrate and visualize.

You might as well know that this system is not child's play. It is work! You cannot do it only when you feel like it, or be sloppy about how you do it. The method is a precise one and works if you will work at it with the self-discipline necessary.

Summary

1. Visualize only what you wish to happen.

2. Repeat it consistently as well as daily.

3. Concentrate and visualize **strongly.** Thought is vibration and a stronger vibration will work better than a weak one.

4. Add color (i.e., think in technicolor) for added vibrational effects.

This is the *general* over-all plan for achieving youth, beauty and health. The *exact formula* for youth and beauty follows.

3.

How to
breathe color
for beauty

Before you begin your color breathing, you should be in a relaxed state. Nearly everyone has tried meditation these days, so, as in meditation, choose a time and place where you will not be interrupted or have any deadlines. Sit in a comfortable position, with spine straight. (If you lie down, you might go to sleep.) You have also heard a lot about biofeedback. To use this terminology, put yourself in an *alpha* state, which means merely to slow down your thinking and breathing to a point where you feel drowsy and couldn't care less what goes on around you. When either in meditation or alpha (both states are similar), wondering what is in the refrigerator for lunch, or thinking about a phone call you intend to make as soon as you are *out,* is not conducive to concentration or best results.

A word about visualization: don't worry about it. If you can imagine, you can visualize. All you need to do to prove to yourself that you can visualize, is to picture the way you looked at some happy time in your life: a graduation, your wedding, a birthday celebration, or whatever. You can recall how joyous you felt and the circumstances which surrounded the occasion. If that doesn't evoke a mental picture, remember when you went to the beach, or the mountains, or your favorite vacation place. The picture will come on strong and that is visualization.

Now that you are relaxed in order to concentrate and visualize, you are ready to begin. Yvonne believes that you should not bite off more than you can chew at one time. "Choose the problem which bothers you most and go to work on that alone," she says, "rather than trying to do everything at once, which only dilutes your progress." As she was telling me this, she showed me how she had begun with a deep wrinkle on one cheek, now as smooth as marble. She said she stretched the wrinkle between her fingers as she looked into the mirror to see how it should look. She demonstrated this to me.

"Next," she said, "decide on a shade of pink; the exact shade is not too important except that it should be a light, rosy and radiant, effervescent pink, not dull or inert looking. You may wish to think of it as pink champagne or a soft pink fire. Take several breaths of this color from anywhere out in front of you for a warm-up. Now breathe in the pink air, this time directing it toward the problem area. *Hold your breath while visualizing the area as you want it to be."* Yvonne visualized her skin smooth and tight where the wrinkle was.

I checked this technique of holding your breath while visualizing the desired condition with Ann Ree Colton, a minister, teacher and expert on spiritual and metaphysical problems. She has proved to be a reliable guide to countless followers for many years, and is revered for her wisdom and kindness. She stated, "If you visualize the desired condition on the holding breath, you are connecting with superconscious energy." This, of course, adds further strength to achieving your desire.

Yvonne uses the color breath on one area three times, before proceeding to the next area. For example, you could begin on a wrinkle on your cheek, then proceed to one under your eye, in whatever order you prefer, putting what is most important to you, first. For added results, you may employ feeling. This can be a feeling of joyousness for future success, or it can be a prayer of gratitude. Yvonne gives thanks between each set of the three color breaths. Ann Ree gives thanks at the end of the total group of breaths. This gratitude is proffered to any unseen helpers, such as angels, helpers, God, or whatever is meaningful to you or your religion. If you hook up to a spiritual power of some kind, it seems to add a leavening just as yeast added to dough causes it to bubble and multiply.

The final step is to put the whole thing out of your

mind and forget it until your next session. "A watched pot never boils."

Summary of the Beauty Color Breathing Formula

1. Adopt a quiet, meditative state of mind.

2. Breathe in pink air from in front of you at eye level for several times. Then breathe in the pink air and mentally direct it to the area you wish to improve. While holding your breath, visualize it as perfect.

3. Do this three times.

4. Feel the joy of accomplishment or offer gratitude for help with that area.

5. Repeat for other areas.

6. Forget about the whole thing until the next session.

Yvonne states that she follows this ritual the first thing upon awakening and the last thing before going to sleep. This is actually an ideal time, since your conscious mind is already sleepy and the drowsy state between waking and sleeping is a natural meditative or *alpha* state. I asked Yvonne if she is lying down at this time and she said yes and admitted that she often falls asleep in the middle of the process. She usually tries to repeat the formula sometime during midday when she can get away by herself and find peace and quiet.

Ann Ree voices one warning: any self-improvement program should not be done for selfishness or vanity, or it may boomerang against you or not work at all! You should make it clear to yourself in the beginning that, as in prayer, you wish to make a change for the good of others as well as yourself. Selfish prayers are not answered as readily as unselfish ones. It is allowable to give pleasure to others by your appearance. Everyone is cheered up when a pretty girl enters a room, but if that pretty girl is self-centered and is obviously using her good looks for personal vanity only, it turns others off. Ask that your improvement be a blessing to others as well as yourself. Or think of it in terms of the Golden Rule. Actually, beauty should be an inner radiance, a spiritual substance which is observed and felt by others. Yvonne believes that one's goal should be to become a good and spiritual individual, and that the color breath for beauty is merely the icing on the cake. Ann Ree agrees. Both women are basically interested in spiritual not personal success.

There is one surprising development which I (Linda) have learned. In programming my etheric, my subconscious mind seems to be listening in and feels the need to get into the act, too. We know that the subconscious is the servant of the conscious mind and does what it is told to do, without reasoning. But I am constantly amazed at how my visualization is picked up by my subconscious as well as by my etheric. I can see the beginnings of the programming of the etheric, when, in addition, suddenly I am the recipient of other visible helps as well. Let us say that I may be working on a smoother skin. I see signs of results from the etheric, but visible helps start rolling in too. I pick up a book and a sentence seems to jump off the page telling how someone else developed a smooth skin. Or someone may tell me about a new skin smoothing cream or I read of a new herbal remedy or nutritional aid. It is definitely past the point of coincidence.

Yvonne states that breathing color has helped some people reduce. I recently learned of one woman who had read *Color Therapy* who lost nine pounds within a few weeks by this method. However, Yvonne has used colors other than pink for reducing, with excellent results. This will be described later.

So don't sell color breathing short. It can work for health as well as beauty!

4.

color breathing
for health

Color breathing has been used successfully for centuries for health purposes. Those who have practiced certain types of yoga, or metaphysics or spiritual healing techniques, etc., consciously or unconsciously, often have used the *color breath* with good results. However, in this book we are not allowed to make any claims for results for two reasons:

    1. The medical monopoly (which is associated with

the drug industry) will not allow it, and

2. Due to individual difference, no two people may get exactly the same results.

I can, however, report what others have experienced. Your body belongs to you and no one can prevent you (so far) from using any treatment you wish. You have nothing to lose and everything to gain from using color. So it is worth a try!

From her own experience Yvonne reports: "About twenty years ago I was told by my doctor that I had no more than five years to live.

I had had a series of light heart attacks; I was suffering from arthritis; I was twenty pounds underweight and completely worn out mentally, emotionally and spiritually. At this time I was running three modeling schools, a household, and raising two children. Business and domestic stresses were weighing heavily on me and I was a wreck. In addition to early wrinkles and bags under my eyes, I also had age (liver) spots on my hands and face.

"Using color breathing cleared my arthritis in one month. All knobs in my body disappeared after using turquoise color breathing for that length of time. My heart returned to normal in approximately six months to a year, due to using pink plus a golden-white color. All of this success was later confirmed by my doctor who didn't know how I had become well. Surprisingly, the liver spots, on which I used pink, took four years to remove.

"My weight also became normal and I am in perfect health today."

But this was not Yvonne's only experience with

color healing. One day, years later, as she was crossing the street, she slipped, fell and broke her leg. When she reached the hospital in great pain, x-rays showed the broken leg was cracked in several places, and both ankles were sprained. The doctor put her leg in a cast and Yvonne insisted on returning home to care for her children. He warned her that, due to her age, she would be in the cast from six weeks to two months, probably longer.

As she described it, "I began to breathe orange to eliminate pain and it worked. I did not need to take the pain killers and tranquilizers the doctor had given me."

As a result of color analysis, and suggestions from color oriented friends, she decided to use a color combination for helping her leg. She used a whitish gray, or mist color for bone mending, added green for nerve strengthening, plus blue for life-force. She mixed these on her mental color palette and then visualized it swathing her entire broken leg, as well as both feet and ankles. She visualized the areas as perfect, accompanied by a firm, silent or audible statement that they were being perfectly healed.

Yvonne reports, "On my next hospital visit the doctor said, 'You really must live right. You're almost ready to come out of the cast. I can't believe it but there it is.' I didn't dare tell him I had been using my own color therapy.

"A week later I shed my cast, which I had worn for only three weeks. I was elated until I noticed my leg was shapeless and discolored. The message came to me intuitively that I was to have faith, and keep breathing color. I did. Now my leg looks as good as the other."

How is color healing done? It may vary with the

individual as well as with the method used. Professionals in any field agree, based on extensive experience: there is *never* only one way to do something. It may be an individual matter since what works for one person may or may not work for another; or the method may be an either/or, or a both/and approach. It is important to understand this concept since various people have reported success in color breathing from different methods. The lesson to be learned here is to study the following methods, all used by *experts* in this field. You may have to experiment until you find what works best for you, which after all, is your own criterion. What feels good to you and what brings results, is your way to success. There are good reasons for these variations: some people have more trouble visualizing than others; concentration comes harder to some; the type of disturbance you are trying to overcome may be more resistant than that of someone else. There are too many variables to expect one plan to suit all, anymore than one type of shoes fits everybody. Choose what appeals to you, and work out your own methods until *you* are satisfied. I am even going to throw in some discoveries of my own which helped me and some others who tried them. If they help you, fine. If not, use your ingenuity to blaze a new trail.

The late Roland T. Hunt, the internationally-known color expert, devised a color method of cleansing his body. I can testify that it works. This method is described in *Man Made Clear for the Nu-Clear Age.*[3]

Like most people who work with color, Roland Hunt was a religious person and asked for Divine help before commencing his routine, and gave thanks after finishing it. Although, in previous books, he described the effects of various colors, in this book *Man Made Clear*, he concentrated on one color for body cleansing of congestion in each area and organ, He named this cleansing process *clarification*, and the single cleansing color, *the light of clarification*, which is a deep violet or medium purple, about the shade of Parma violets. (See violet in color chart on back cover.)

He stated that the persistent beaming of this color on various parts of the body dissolved congestion from a solid to a fluid state and that within twenty-four hours after the clarification, there might well be a feeling of discomfort while the toxins were being discharged from the body. This might include sinus discharge, kidney or intestinal activity, even underarm perspiration with an unpleasant odor, all of which should be welcome, he said, because the body was ridding itself of undesirable toxins. He felt that nerves, circulation and other unresolved pressures of many kinds benefited from this cleansing process. Here was his method:

Beginning at the top of the head and holding his palms facing downward toward the crown of the head, he would visualize a beam of this deep violet light from his palms focusing on the various glands located in the head: the pituitary, pineal, hypothalamus, thalamus and others. He held his palms about nine inches away from the area to be treated, he said. If there were congestion here or elsewhere, one would note resistance in the palms which would feel warm. When the resistance melted, he said the palms should feel cool, signaling that it was time to move on to the next station. (I found that three inches, instead of nine worked best for me, and that heat appeared in the area being treated, not in my palms.)

Regardless of the position of his hands, *he* always held them about nine inches from the area to be treated, and always visualized the deep violet color streaming through his palms to the area being treated.

The next placement of his hands, after finishing the crown of the head, was to place his left hand in front of his brow, and his right hand directly behind it at the back of his head.

He then moved his left hand to the bridge of the nose and his right hand to the base of the brain.

The next position was putting one hand, each, beside the level of the ears and the parotid glands. He stated that an ear discharge might result.

The next placement was on the sides of the neck, over the carotid and lymph glands, for emotional and blood pressure balance. (See anatomy chart.)

Next: he placed his left hand over the thyroid and parathyroid (in the front of the neck) and the right hand over the occiput at the back of the neck where the head joins the neck.

Next, he placed both hands fairly close together over the lungs, then the right hand over the thymus (see anatomy chart), then the heart.

Next, he lowered his hands over the digestive organs, the liver, gall bladder, pancreas and spleen, later over the intestines and colon.

Finally, reaching behind him he placed one hand over each kidney, in the small of the back, and the adrenals which lie atop of each kidney.

Roland Hunt stated that this procedure might take as long as forty minutes and should not be done oftener than every other day.

Yvonne's method is related to, though different from, Roland Hunt's and yet she was unaware of his book at the time she formulated her approach. She breathes exactly as she does for the beauty routine, but merely uses different colors. First, if an area of the body is causing trouble, she visually floods it with a pinkish orange. (See color chart on back cover.) She describes this color as a soft, apricot-orange. On the holding breath, after inhaling the color, she holds the orange where it is needed if there is pain (as described earlier in the account of her leg fracture) or if no pain is present, merely to wake up the cells to activate them. After this, she applies a deep violet to cleanse the cells in the disturbed area. She follows this with the color needed for healing of the condition described in the next chapter.

Ann Ree Colton uses the Yoga method as follows:

She focuses the color necessary on the area to be healed and breathes through her nose, with her mouth closed. She inhales slowly and rhythmically to the count of five, holds the breath to the count of ten, during which time she visualizes the area needing healing as perfect; then exhales to the count of five. She repeats this cycle five times, giving thanks at the end *knowing* that the healing is being done. She says that this series of five cycles should be done only once daily.

Ann Ree states that this method stimulates the 72,000 Nadis, or acupuncture points, in the body.

Yvonne does her method three times, once upon waking, once midday, and the last on retiring. She breathes color only three times each session, as in her beauty routine. If she uses orange, then violet, then the healing color, this totals nine breaths.

I developed my own method, for what it is worth, and by using it I grew a complete head of new hair!

Someone had taught me what is known in yoga, as the complete breath.[4] This is done by inhaling, during which time the stomach balloons outward. While holding this outward position, I mentally visualize the breath going upward to and expanding the lungs, completely filling them. If you are going to use this breath for treating, as the yogis do, you do it at this point, as I will explain later, then as you exhale, pull the stomach in. To check yourself to see if you are doing this breath correctly, you put one hand on your stomach or lower abdomen, the other on your lungs. As you inhale, the hand on the stomach should rise as the stomach distends. The hand on the lungs remains quiet, since the air expands the lungs internally and *sideways*, without rising upward. When you exhale, the hand on your abdomen goes inward with it. Later, you can direct the breath elsewhere in your body.

Now about my hair: Normally, my hair has always been thick, but recently, as with millions of other people, it began to fall alarmingly. This may be due to radioactivity in the air, or smog. It cannot be diet in my case, since as a nutrition researcher my diet is better than average. I receive letters by the hundreds from panicky men and women asking for an explanation of and help for falling hair. The answers are found in two of my books, *Secrets of Health and Beauty*[5] and *Beauty Questions and Answers*[6].

I can also use external helps, of course, but since I was at work on research for this book at the time my hair fall became noticeable, I decided to see what color breathing could do.

Every morning during meditation (once daily) I used the complete breath, which I mentally colored golden as used by others for general healing purposes, and carried it mentally from my lungs upward to my scalp. I mentally held it there and affirmed either audibly or silently, "This healing breath is now stimulating a thick growth of hair on my head." I held it there for a short while. If I ran out of breath, I breathed again, and, like Yvonne, repeated it for a third time. To my astonishment, somewhere along the way between the second and third breath my head became very warm. As someone has pointed out, circulation follows attention. At any rate, I knew something was happening and gave thanks. Later at the same sitting I also used the pink breath for beautiful, thick hair, then turned my mind off the whole subject.

I did not keep track of how long it took, but several weeks later, I discovered a short bristling stubble forming on my scalp at the base of the longer hairs. That growth has now reached about an inch in length and a new, second bristle has begun! I became so excited, I also began using external measures, as well, to speed things up, as described in *Beauty Questions and Answers*.

But after this, something still more peculiar began to happen. After leaving my scalp, I took a new breath and carried it to other parts of my body. There, too, if I waited long enough the area became warm, and I knew I had made contact. But although I had been using the golden healing breath as usual, occasionally, on an organ, the gold would change of its own accord to another color: green, violet, or whatever.

I questioned Ann Ree about this and she listened without surprise. She said, "Color is a chameleon. The color you saw develop at certain areas was being given you because that organ needed the frequency of that particular color at that time for healing or improvement."

Even Yvonne, when I later told her about it, seemed unimpressed. She agreed that we often make our own colors and shades of those colors as needed. She had had the same experience.

I have one more tip which may help you as it helped me. In concentrating on the golden healing color going from area to area on my own body, I often found that my attention wandered. So I devised a method to keep it under control. I visualized the golden healing color as coming from a spot light which I mentally held in my hand, or actually held my right hand above the problem spot, visualizing the needed color as radiating from the palm, and focused on whichever area I wished, holding it there until time to move it to the next area. Even so, if another color was needed, it made its appearance (and more quickly) under the play of light from the imaginary spotlight or palm, because I was able to keep my attention riveted on the area rather than having it wander off out the window or elsewhere.

These explanations indicate that we may need different props to hold us on course.

If you wake up in the middle of the night and have trouble going back to sleep, don't fret. Get to work on your color breathing. You will not only be doing your body a favor, you will also no doubt promptly fall asleep again.

In the next chapter, you will learn more about what colors to use for which disturbances.

5.

COLORS FOR
VARIOUS PROBLEMS

We make no claims in this chapter for healing. Results which have taken place are merely reported. The medical profession would like you to check with your doctor when in doubt or in need of treatment.

You can learn to use certain colors for certain conditions as practiced centuries ago by the priests of Egypt, and other early cultures. By learning how to breathe color, you can direct it, together with a source of life energy contained in breath, to any part of your body, hopefully giving your glands, your organs, even your face and eyes a tune-up. Improved health, youth and beauty have resulted by breathing correctly with color.

What colors are best for certain conditions?

The entire color picture has not yet been clarified. Bits and pieces are falling into place, and you may make some discoveries of your own. Some long held suppositions also appear to be changing. For example, as explained in *Color Therapy* (to which this book is in a sense a sequel) you will notice that with equipment, such as lamps, panes of glass for filtering the sun, etc., *exact* shades including certain color frequencies and wave lengths were recommended.

Yvonne, on the other hand, feels that the colors used in color breathing need not be exact because there is no light to dilute them and because color breathing may help us adjust our own colors for our own conditions as we need them. They can *come to us* as we ask for help. The colors which Yvonne has used are more pastel in form than the deeper jewel tones recommended in *Color Therapy*. (See color chart on back cover.)

Another recent report came our way via a color therapist who said that new information is being received through some clairvoyants; i.e., colors long considered traditional for certain problems, may not be a wise selection after all. White light, she reported, is an example.

This may come as a shock for those who have used white light for everything. It does indeed contain all colors and has long been considered *tried and true*, a catchall or panacea for almost everything, including healing. White light has always been associated by spiritual healers with the Christ light and considered impervious, which is still true. However, according to our informant, the white light may be too dazzling and too high in vibration for some people; therefore it should be reserved for protection purposes only. For example, if speakers mentally surround themselves with the white light as they stand on the platform, they may repel, rather than endear those in the audience whose vibrations are lower. To promote a feeling of rapport, it might be better to use the rosy pink of love around you and your audience, as practiced by the Rosicrucians.

One man stated that because he is a dowser and his subject controversial, he is often met by stoney resistance from some members of the audience as he steps to the platform to begin his lecture. When we asked him what he did about it, he said, "I just surround the audience as well as myself with the pink color of Divine love, and everybody seems to relax and be in a more receptive mood. At least they can then judge for themselves instead of being influenced by preconceived bias against my subject."

On the other hand, there is no substitute for the white light for protection purposes. Many people cleanse their entire house morning and night by visualizing each room filled with white light. This procedure is simultaneously combined with speaking the name of Jesus Christ, a powerful defender, since the vibration of the name alone is impenetrable. People state that when they surround their house and property with white light daily their premises have, to date, been protected from vandalism. Mrs. Eleanore Thedick stated that the effect would last eight hours.

One man also told us about two people who came to

his house one day and became more and more restless. Finally one of them blurted out, "We cannot stay in this house any longer. We are acutely uncomfortable." After they left the man learned that these two had been dabbling in black magic and did not know that he routinely cleansed his house and property with white light twice daily. The vibration was too much for them. They had actually felt it!

Personal property can be protected in the same way. A friend, another clairvoyant (we attract them like flies) knitted some slippers for an acquaintance and mailed them to her, blessing them with white light as she sent them. The slippers apparently never arrived at the RFD mailbox address as directed on the label—at least the acquaintance did not receive them.

Two months later a neighbor found the slippers under a bush, covered with leaves and twigs, but otherwise unharmed. The vandal who had taken them from the mailbox had apparently opened the package, and finding the slippers *too hot to handle* dropped them under a bush and ran. The wrapping was recovered under another bush. The clairvoyant who had made the slippers later *read* this story which came to her. She claimed that she still saw the light around the slippers.

Meanwhile, people who have previously used white for healing, may try gold instead. More and more reports are accumulating that it may be *the* healing color when a specific color for a condition is unknown.

One color worker does not bother with individual colors at all. She mentally breathes and visualizes a rainbow around her and assumes that the body will choose from it the color *it* needs for its well-being.

The following colors are those used by *Yvonne* in her work with color breathing for various conditions:

Pink Breath: for wrinkles, acne, sagginess, puffiness, crepiness and looseness of the skin anywhere on face or body.

Turquoise breath: blue-green has created changes in the circulatory system. Has relieved respiratory ailment, arthritis, some heart and gastric conditions. Has removed excess fat when alternated with pink; also used to increase weight. Yvonne says to use turquoise three times, then pink three times, but visualize the desired outline of the body in pink. (The turquoise is used internally, the pink externally).

Orange: a soft, apricot-orange containing some pink removes pain, but does not cure it.

Dark blue: tinged with green, or green with a blue tinge accompanied by an opaque film for mending bones.

Sky blue: has improved memory, intellectual or artistic talents. Also used for a feeling of relaxation or well being.

Dark green: to purify the blood and for any associated diseases.

Grass green: for success, monetary gain, acquisition of possessions, **providing** it is qualified with the statements, "according to the will of the Father." This must not be used for something illegal or which belongs to someone else. There is enough for all. Claim your own share; but the claim must never conflict with God's laws. Yvonne advises: spend at least five minutes morning and night seeing yourself surrounded with this color, and emotionally experience the desired result of what you wish or need. Repeat three times together with prayers as mentioned above,

Pale green: has improved vision, eye injuries, or diseases, unless involved with circulation, nerves, etc., in which case the desired color for these conditions is used. According to

49

Yvonne, send the pale green breath first to the solar plexus, then up to the eyes, Repeat three times. Couple with statement of desired condition, prayers, followed by thanks, as usual.

Medium green: for individual characteristics; to change personality for the better, eliminate bad habits, acquire new habits. Breathe in the medium green, sending it first to the solar plexus, then transfer to heart and head areas at least three times in each area. Accompany it with a picture of yourself as you wish to be: the new personality. This will require six breaths total at each session.

Purple breath: a cleansing breath for both physical and emotional disturbances. If conditions of danger of any kind, or if negative conditions are present, visualize the purple light beginning from your feet and working upward, enveloping your entire body, while asking that any danger or disturbance be eliminated according to God's will. Then immediately follow by drawing around you from head to toe, a white light or cocoon to insulate you and maintain your protection. A marvelous help in driving, flying, or other hazardous experiences.

Pale orchid: for spiritual attunement.

Deep pinkish rose: for creating loving rapport with others. Also has been used for regeneration of organs.

Gold: a general, overall healing color to irradiate you from head to toe. Also considered helpful for inner head problems, growths, etc. When in doubt as to what color to use for healing, try gold.

In addition, Yvonne uses these colors for the following disturbances:

Bones: teal blue (a blue-green shade deeper than turquoise)
Nerves: golden white plus leaf green

Anemia: dark green

Muscles: pink

Insomnia: lavender or blue

Yvonne has made new discoveries along the way. One, previously mentioned, is to apply the apricot-orange shade to the area needing help, at the same time commanding the cells of the area to wake up and start functioning. Talking to the body is described in *Help Yourself to Health.* Deep violet for cleansing is used next, followed by the color needed for the condition.

Another innovation came to Yvonne in a dream. This is an imaginary skullcap to be worn either at night or applied immediately upon wakening in the morning. It is mentally applied by visualization to the body and face, covered by a crystal-like covering of pink like a second skin. The cap apparently is meant to be magnetic, according to the dream. Strings of light are visualized as pulling inwardly on any and all areas which seem to have lost muscle tone, or firmness in face or figure. This would apply to drooping face muscles, eyelids, or wherever else you need help. As you visualize these areas attached to the magnetic strings, Yvonne says, "You can actually feel the inner pull."

If any descriptions of using color do not seem clear to you, don't worry about it. Work out your own method. It may work best for you.

6.

RESULTS of
COLOR bREATHiNG

Yvonne gives further details of how she breathed pink for her own beauty problems. She says, "After erasing the wrinkle on my left cheek, which took eight to nine months, though I noticed improvement within a month, it took only two months to remove sagging, crepiness, wrinkles, etc., from my neck; three months from my forehead. The most difficult area in my face was around my eyes. I have a tendency to dark circles, although the bags are gone.

In fact, I am still working on my eyes. The upper eye lids are now as I want them.

"I have rearranged my weight, improved the contours of my face and body and have removed all stretch marks from having three children. I had my last child at forty-three, an age when the skin is supposed to have lost its elasticity, and is considered unable to bounce back to its original youthful condition."

Several students in Yvonne's classes state that they have had luck in taking off weight especially in the leg area, as well as eliminating gastric attacks and relieving arthritis, all with the turquoise breath.

One of Yvonne's models wrote her:

I have to let the world know what a miracle breathing turquoise has done for me.

My problem of excess weight in my legs has, as you know, been completely removed in two short weeks by breathing turquoise, thereby enabling me to again be one of your successful bathing suit models. I will never be able to thank you enough.

Yvonne states that when she, herself, feels depressed, she inhales turquoise, sending the breath to her toes and finger tips, coursing through her entire body, then up the spinal cord into her head, ending with a shower of a blue-green air splashing all around her.

Yvonne is determined that for success, any visualization must also be accompanied by a firm silent or audible statement of what you wish to achieve. For example, in this case, one might say, while visualizing the turquoise color at work, "I am becoming cheerful and happy." (Do not mention what you are trying to get rid of.)

Another of Yvonne's students wrote her:

Remember me? I am the one who twisted my knee wrong getting out of a chair, leaving me unable to straighten my leg out.

As I told you when I first spoke to you, it was quite painful and having to walk with the knee bent didn't look too great. I tried heat, massage, etc., but nothing helped.

After breathing orange as you told me, my knee is back to normal and it took only one evening.

I'm most grateful.

Yvonne tells the next story.

"One day as I was eating lunch in one of my town's little coffee shops, a bespectacled, middle-aged business man I had known for years came up and asked if he could sit with me. Naturally I said yes, but wondered why he asked, since he had never said more than "Hello" to me in fifteen years.

"He started the conversation by complimenting me about my modeling school, and 'youthology' (Yvonne's metaphysical approach to youth and beauty) plus color breathing which I teach there, and then asked whether I could give him a suggestion or two to restore to him, as he put it the 'vim and vigor of a young man.' I could tell by his slight embarrassment that he didn't know quite how to go about asking for help. I briefly outlined the procedure of color breathing, then suggested that he breathe in a deep shade of rose, sending the breath and the color to the area needing help. I told him to visualize himself as being virile while holding the breath only as long as comfortable, then allowing it to rise, mentally, up the spinal cord, leaving the color there, then dismissing the whole thing from his mind. I suggested, of course, that he follow this technique morning and night, and any other times convenient.

"After another cup of coffee, I said I had to get back to my classes. He also had to get back to his business, he said, and we went our respective ways. I never gave the incident another thought.

"A couple of weeks later, he passed me by chance on the street and came up hurriedly and said, 'Yvonne, I have been meaning to come to your studio to thank you. You must be a genius or something.'

"I said, 'It evidently worked, huh?'

"Like a charm,' he answered. He added that he felt like a new man; his whole life had changed. Even his business had picked up.

"This same change has taken place in other men and women who have started to breathe rose. A woman in her early forties, came to me one day for help. She was fat, dowdy, crabby and thoroughly disenchanted with herself, her husband, marriage, and life in general. She had heard about color breathing, and wondered if it would help her.

"I did not know exactly what she wanted: a change in her looks, health, husband, or perhaps all three. It turned out that the real problem was that she wasn't too desirable, which her husband had told her several times. But the sad part was that she herself no longer desired physical love.

And that was what was really bothering her.

"I first told her to start thinking kinder thoughts about her husband as well as mentally wrapping him in a cloud of rose, as if it were connecting her heart with his heart. Then I suggested that she take a warm bath before bedtime, visualize herself reliving the feeling of being a newlywed, and see herself feel responsive while she enveloped the pelvic area with rose air. I assured her that she should soon feel a difference.

"When I saw her next I thought I noticed a new bounce in her walk, but neither of us mentioned her problem. She seemed a little less crabby and grumpy, but I figured maybe it was just my imagination.

"About a month later, she approached me secretively and said, 'Yvonne, breathing rose is great. I feel like a young girl again and my husband thinks I'm beautiful."

Yvonne concludes, "Thinking color plus galvanizing emotion for good and positive results, is what *really* makes it so."

Another example involved a couple who had been married for thirty years without having children, which they longed for. They had been to doctors, taken various medical treatments. None had helped. The doctors told them flatly that it was too late; they were too old.

As a last resort they asked Yvonne if she could help. To the man, Yvonne suggested that he breathe a deep rose shade, and visualize himself as virile and deeply in love with his wife, which he already was. To the woman, Yvonne suggested that she breathe rose and direct the breath plus the color to her reproductive organs, simultaneously imagining how it must feel to be pregnant. Yvonne also recommended that the woman read a book on motherhood and sent her to infant shops in department stores to get the feeling of being an expectant mother. Yvonne suggested that they sit together and mentally wrap themselves in a cloud of rose, alternating with pink.

Six months later the couple told Yvonne that the wife was pregnant. Eventually they had a baby girl.

Here are two letters, among others, which came to me recently. One read:

> A friend of mine gave me your book **Color Therapy.** I am really enjoying it. I find since I am breathing pink, so many nice things are coming to me, including a lot of them pink. For example, my neighbor gives me beautiful bouquets of pink flowers which cheer me up. Thank you for writing your book. It helps to escape the sad world of today.

Another reader wrote:

> I read your book **Color Therapy.** I have been using color therapy on myself with light treatments as well as in my clothing for some time. Now I am planning to make a color therapy room in our haymow!

Nothing is impossible!

7.

MORE HELP WITH COLOR BREATHING

Color breathing is a new, growing art and all of the information is not yet in. Although we cannot answer your letters due to our extremely crowded schedules, we would be delighted to hear of your discoveries as you, too, work with color breathing. You may make a helpful discovery or have an important contribution to share. If so, please address us in care of the publisher. In so doing, you may help the growth of this new art.

Yvonne has already shared her experiences, and many have benefited. At the last minute, just before this book was "put to bed," we received news about another researcher in color breathing. This information appeared in a small out-of-print booklet, loaned to us by a friend who collects color therapy books. It was written by the late Ivah Bergh Whitten, a former co-worker with Roland T. Hunt, the internationally famous writer on color (now deceased).

The booklet by Mrs. Whitten, called *Colour Breathing*, was published in 1948 by the C. W. Daniel Company, Ltd., in England, but is apparently out of print. However, we will include the highlights so that you, too, can benefit from this tiny, but important, booklet.

Mrs. Whitten, an Englishwoman, was a lecturer and teacher of color breathing to students in fourteen different countries. She was, apparently, also a highly spiritual woman who worked with the ascended masters from which she says she derived her information. (Remember, we are *reporting*, not evaluating, what appears in the booklet.)

Her colors differ slightly, in some instances, from the ones others use. For example, here are the pinks she labels for certain purposes:

American beauty pink or old rose: sex
Clear shell pink: creative love and tolerance
Soft salmon pink: universal love, love for all humanity, self-sacrificing mother love

She does not mention a pink for wrinkles, but has another approach to skin, which she calls not only *color* breathing but *skin* breathing. She states that according to dermatologists, wrinkles are the result of a deep clogging of the skin with impurities which can be removed by color breathing. Before giving you the colors she suggests for skin breathing, it is important to understand *how* she does skin or color breathing.

She explains. "The entire process of colour breathing is in an upward circular direction, starting with the feet, ending above the head in a brilliant swirl of colour. Acting as a skin function, skin colour breathing serves to free the surfaces in a rapidly rising circular path as you inhale, then as you exhale it comes through the pores of the skin outward, carrying all before it as it neutralizes or removes residual poisons. To do this treatment, she says, "From your feet, your colour breathing should rise in a circular path beneath your skin surface, up your legs, up your thighs, about the buttocks, abdomen, and the entire torso to the throat. Then lift your arms high and release it in a spiral whirl of colour."

She adds, "It is not easy to accomplish at first, but may be acquired only through persistent efforts, and is well worth the effort.

"Never, under any circumstances, strain your lungs! The attention must be centered first on visualization, which must be vivid. To this you add colour. Always remember that colour is a potent, powerful force and must be used with great discrimination just as you would use electricity or any other great force.

"Place your physical body in tune with your Divine, higher self. Once you have accomplished this union, colour breathing will do the rest."

Mrs. Whitten not only firmly believes this method of skin color breathing eliminates the clogging substances in the skin which lead to wrinkles, she goes even further: she believes that the texture of your skin is a give away to the type of thinking you do: spiritual, or materialistic; joyful or depressed; unselfish or selfish; loving or hate-filled and resentful. In fact, she states that *any* negative thought you consistently entertain *must* be dissolved inwardly before you can expect outward success and beauty. If you make a practice of keeping your thoughts joyful, poised, serene, tolerant and loving, letting joy radiate from within you, she says, you will achieve outer as well as inner beauty. If, on the other hand, you dwell upon negative thought forms, you will not get the desired results. She feels that color breathing will help you clear the way. You do this by choosing the *opposite* color from your negative mood.

For example, she says if you are feeling irritable you are probably unconsciously generating an angry red. If, instead, you surround yourself with the quietness of its opposite color, blue, you will neutralize the irritability. She believes a rich delft blue, the color of serenity, may help those with high blood pressure due to irritation with small inconsequential happenings. She considers jade green a color of tact and diplomacy. So if you are about to blow your top at someone, think blue, followed by jade green instead!

This color symbology becomes more and more fascinating. Mrs. Whitten considers dull brown the color of selfishness; golden brown a color of conservation. For example, she says, "A man who is afraid to face life in a suit of grey (which she believes denotes a fear complex) may become positively dynamic in a suit of rich deep blue or golden brown.

"I put one man," she continues, "with a 'fear complex' and a grey suit into a tweed suit of English heather colours and he became a success. He insisted, however, that the change was due to his tie, which was green, the colour of finance.

"Another man gave up profanity when he gave up his red ties!"

Mrs. Whitten also reunited a mother and daughter after years of estrangement, when they both studied color and the mother gave up her "favorite" grey of fear, and the daughter stopped wearing the dull brown of selfishness. Both "learned the value of the soft salmon pink of unselfish or Universal Love," and the estrangement ended.

This brings up two possible questions: These changes were made in clothing. Would color breathing be as effective? The late Dr. Oscar Brunler (*Color Therapy*) answers, "Visualizing color will bring the same results as actual color. Whatever affects our mind, affects our body."

The other question is: Doesn't your own favorite color provide an automatic correct selection of color? Mrs. Whitten answers, *no!* Your favorite color *may* be safe, but it *might* be keyed to an objectionable complex, in which case its persistent use may fasten the complex more permanently in your consciousness. Mrs. Whitten states that choosing a color representing the opposite trait will neutralize the unwanted complex. For example: Mrs. Whitten recommends the pink of Universal Love to dissolve the fear complex which is represented by grey. (Information in

Color Therapy will give you further help; the meaning of each color is explained.) In general, beware of black, dull browns, grey, muddy colors, and the deep angry reds. (Flame red with some yellow in it is apparently acceptable, since it often shows up in healers.)

But the most exciting information from Mrs. Whitten is yet to come. She suggests there are certain colors which are best, though not for everybody, in achieving health or beauty of skin and body, but *for each separate individual*. In other words, she believes, when it comes to our bodies, that like our finger prints, our colors also differ from others. She was apparently told by "the people upstairs" as Hans Holzer,[7] calls our unseen helpers, that each person has his own soul color, but is often entirely unaware of what it is. Thus he goes bumbling through life like a round peg in a square hole lacking success, accomplishment and even health.

Mrs. Whitten states categorically, "All things with which you deal, or come in productive contact with, must in a very direct manner be keyed to your *own* soul colour. Otherwise the result may be discord and failure. The key to your success and accomplishment is this knowledge (of your soul colour) linked to intelligent effort." She says, "It will unlock life's door to success and all necessary supply, at least in knowledge, if not in actual money. Each person has his individualized soul colour which, harmonized with his individualized source of expression as well as supply, can be contacted only through these channels. Any attempts by other means (no matter how fine the motive) will fail to produce results for you. Others may benefit by your efforts, but you may always lack!"

Mrs. Whitten continues, "On the other hand, if you are linked up to and are using your soul colour, its sphere of usefulness seems limitless. I have personally seen it cause the helpless to walk, the dumb to speak, the deaf to hear, and those who have given up to rally and take up new lives of usefulness."

In a companion booklet, *What Colour Means to You*, written by the same author and published by the same publisher, Mrs. Whitten says that while your soul color is the real "You" and is your first consideration, we also have three other colors of importance: our *color of inspiration, color of activity, and color of rest*. She advises surrounding yourself mentally with your inspirational color during meditation (she calls this color of inspiration "your private telephone number to your higher self.") She recommends mentally visualizing your color of rest when you are weary. She states that by so doing, you can achieve in twenty minutes restoration for tired nerves and a fagged body which would ordinarily require two hours of regular rest or relaxation, and she states that surrounded with your color of activity during your work periods no other person can separate you from your perfect plan of success and achievement.

So she urges us all to learn our soul, inspirational, activity and rest color to harmonize our lives.

With that dramatic announcement, she abruptly changes the subject without telling us *how* to find these important colors. Perhaps she meant to cover them in another book, but if so, we couldn't find it; or maybe she never got around to it. So we were thrown upon our own resources and had to do some scrambling to learn the answers. Four of us got busy, pooled our knowledge and found our colors! Here's how:

Metaphysics teaches that if you want the answer to a problem, ask for it three nights in a row, just before going to sleep, and the answer will come. You may specify contact with your higher self, your subconscious mind, or "the people upstairs." You may ask for the information in a dream, or just ask, period. Many inventors use this method with great success. If you do not dream, or stipulate that method, you will probably be walking or driving down the street a day or so later or be involved in a simple household chore and the answer will come out of the blue. Some people wake up with the answer. Whatever the method, it works. Thousands of people have testified to this. And the answer is always valid, they report. Two of us, including me, used this asking method to find our soul color. Since I witnessed mine first hand, I will tell you how it happened. But first, I must tell you that all my life I have had a favorite color, without which I feel I cannot live. It is so evident in the furnishings of my house and the choice of my clothes, that it is no secret: it is turquoise. But I also like blues in all shades. Green is O.K., but doesn't necessarily turn me on. But combine the blues and green into turquoise or a related color, and I light up like a torch! So when I began to hunt for my soul color, I was sure it would be turquoise. Edgar Cayce had told me it was the color of my aura (others had seen it, too) and he said that usually one's favorite color was the basic aura color. So before I asked the first night, I was sure it would be turquoise. But it wasn't and was I surprised!

The answer came in a dream the very first night. In the dream I was shown a poem in print. I do not know what all the words were. All my eyes seemed to be glued to were the first three words which read, "It is better." Knowing that dreams come in symbols, I wondered what in the world this meant. As I watched those three words, suddenly one of the words changed so that the sentence now read, "It is butter!" End of dream. So my soul color is apparently yellow! And know what? I am not particularly fond of yellow. But I am stuck with it and using it every way possible, even trying it instead of pink for wrinkles. It is too soon to see results, but yellow certainly feels good to me. I don't have to fight to remember or visualize it; it just seems to come naturally into my mind's eye.

The others who joined the experiment of finding their soul color agree. Each of our soul colors are different, but somehow we feel at ease with them, and it is a natural feeling; nothing forced. I found my other colors by a different method, which I will describe shortly. My inspirational color turned out to be turquoise! The activity color, green, and the rest color, blue. These click with me, as the others found that their "secondary" colors clicked with them, too.

One night I must have been questioning that butter-yellow dream without realizing it. So I had a second dream. I saw a yellow gate, and a sign which read, "This opens everything," (for me, that is), so I no longer doubt.

If you use the asking method, unless you stipulate a dream, don't try to program when or how you will receive the answer. Just relax, forget about it. It *will* come. Or you can use the following method as two of the group did to find all four of their colors. I used it to find my secondary colors. This was by means of the pendulum. Don't gasp. If you know how to handle a pendulum, you have a handy little ally. But you *must* follow the rules to the letter or it becomes a farce.

I have covered the use of the pendulum in depth in my book, *Get Well Naturally*,[8] in the chapter, "Do-It-Yourself Radiesthesia" but I will repeat the highlights here so that you can get right to work.

The pendulum should be treated with respect. It is not just a crazy toy; it should not be used for parlor games, or for picking winning horses, or trying to beat the stock market.

Instead, it is a form of dowsing, or a small geiger counter. Its use is limited to "yes" and "no" answers. So don't expect it to compute a complex problem for you. It won't.

The pendulum is not as "far out" as you may think. It is used at least by two well known psychologists for therapy work, by one laboratory technician for testing food and water, and by many others for various purposes.

It has been used for thousands of years and people who have become expert with it get some astounding information, unavailable by other means, or sometimes confirming it. One man, a chemical engineer with several university degrees and a longtime membership in the American Society of Dowsers, considers it standard equipment in his business. "But," he warns, "you must *always* pray before asking the question you wish answered, so that you will contact the 'right' source, and not a fly-by-night-spirit or someone else's subconscious mind. Otherwise the pendulum becomes no more reliable than a ouija board, which can lead you astray." (Further information is given in

Help Yourself to Health.)

Mrs. Whitten wrote that your soul color would be one of seven, each one related to the notes in the musical scale:

1. Red—musical note C
2. Orange—musical note D
3. Yellow—musical note E
4. Green—musical note F

5. Blue—musical note G
6. Indigo—musical note A
7. Violet—musical note B

If you are going to use the pendulum to ascertain your soul color, use this list of seven colors. (I added turquoise to my list. Actually it is a blend of two colors, blue and green, not one alone.)

You can buy a pendulum (see Books n' Things) or you can make one by tying a six to eight inch thread on a large-ish bead (preferably not metal) on one end and a smaller bead on the other end so the thread won't slip from your fingers. If you are right handed, hold the pendulum in your right hand. If you are left handed, use your left. You may, or need not, rest your elbow on a table while you hold the pendulum.

After praying for Divine guidance in answering your question, mentally ask the question, "Is this my soul color?" With the opposite hand you may point with a pencil to each color in turn as you ask the question. If the answer is *yes,* the pendulum should turn of its own accord in a clockwise circle. If the answer is *no*, it should revolve in a counter-clockwise direction. If it does not move at all, you have not yet made contact with the correct source of guidance. If it oscillates from side to side, you have asked the wrong question and need to rephrase it.

When people start to use a pendulum for the first time, it may not budge. Men seem to have more trouble than women. Perhaps it is because they are less intuitive, although there are some high-powered successful male pendulum users.

In any case, keep your mind a blank so that you will not influence the pendulum's answer. It can be influenced by your own strong thinking. Avoid this by remaining perfectly neutral. If you begin to get answers, continue. Find out your inspirational, activity and rest colors, too. Do not work more than about ten to fifteen minutes at a time. And drink no alcohol before using a pendulum!

If no answer comes at first, put the pendulum in a small box or container and wait until another time. No one else should ever use your pendulum, which soon becomes imbued with your own vibration. Eventually, as you become more relaxed with the pendulum, it will respond and become more proficient.

Mrs. Whitten says that if your soul color turns out to be one of the first four on the list of seven, "You should recuperate more quickly from illness or overstrain by visualizing and drawing up the energy colour from the earth's surface, through the soles of your feet, up the base of your spine, and upward." (You need not stand up, however; you may lie down during visualizing.)

"If your soul colour turns out to be one of the last

three, you should draw the energy from above, downward through your head, body and eventually to your feet," she concludes.

Whether you follow this method, or the ones we have discussed earlier in the book, check the anatomy charts first. Become acquainted with your body. You can mentally draw the color toward the part of your body needing improvement, still inhaling as you do, and stating and visualizing the desired results on the holding breath, giving thanks when you have finished.

On learning Mrs. Whitten's method, at first I brought my soul color through the soles of my feet upward, stopping along the way mentally at various points of my body to "treat" areas needing help. Then I decided to return to my earlier method. I drew in and filled my entire body with my soul color first, then, via the total or complete breath (page 40) I distributed it to the areas where it was needed, inhaling a fresh supply of the color to each new area and on the holding breath stated and visualized my desire. I like this better because for me the area becomes warm almost immediately (although it took time at first). When the area has warmed, I know the energy has arrived to do its work. Since Mrs. Whitten is not here to teach us her method, we will have to experiment until we find what is best for each of us.

In any case, however you do it, the *final* step may be an overall visualization on the holding breath as you state silently or aloud, "I am now radiantly healthy, youthful and beautiful (or handsome if you are a man)."

Then, since real beauty comes from within, it is time to share our blessings with others. We should draw the

Universal Love color of soft salmon pink from above, through our heads into our body, hold briefly, and then radiate it outward lovingly to others. Everyone in this world, whether they realize it or not, needs all the Divine love they can get. As a result your own inner beauty will shine through, and your skin texture will reflect it.

But this should not be a selfish goal. You have already had your own treatment. Now share your blessings and Divine love with others. In addition to radiating the salmon pink lovingly toward them, actually feel that love, and smile! I have written elsewhere that the easiest face lift is a smile. But smile not only with your lips, but with your eyes and your voice, to extend the love toward your recipient.

If you truly try to do this to lighten the load of others, not to embellish yourself, you will begin to generate an inner shining beauty which you cannot buy in a jar!

8.

COLOR
iN
ACTiON

As you grow spiritually and work with color—which may be an outgrowth of spiritual development—unexplained experiences may happen to you. Various people have come to me to report some new, inexplicable occurrence. As long as you are not dabbling in psychic or spiritualistic or black magic fields, and keep yourself constantly protected with the white light, there is no danger. Even so, some people have been bewildered, some confused, others frightened at unexplained experiences. Men as well as women have actually questioned their sanity in some cases, as Yvonne did when she saw her "pink star" vision.

One man, close to fifty, a Ph.D. on the faculty of a large and outstanding Eastern university, had had a prolonged religious background, including doing some missionary work in foreign countries. He is now teaching a down-to-earth subject, entirely unconnected with anything spiritual or religious. He has also been exposed to much suffering in various channels. Suddenly he began having premonitive dreams which came true and acted as guides to help himself and others. He came to me in great concern, and I, in turn, referred him to a spiritual teacher who knows much more than I about such subjects. She pronounced that he was indeed opening up spiritually with surprising speed, a fact confirmed by his spiritual-type dreams, on which she is an expert.

An increasing number of people are also seeing auras, those colors which surround each person and vary according to their health, vitality, thoughts, and possible spiritual growth. Most people do not see auras, while others yearn to see them. I belong to the latter group. Occasionally I run across instructions which explain how to learn to see auras, but somehow, I believe that this is something which should not be forced. Just as "when the student is ready, the teacher will appear," I believe that when a person is spiritually ready, the auras will become visible.

I will never forget the time when, years ago, Adelle Davis, the unpredictable, arrived at my house one day in great excitement. She grabbed me by the hand, rushed me into a room, pulled down the shades to produce darkness,

74

shoved me into a chair, saying, "I have brought a pair of special glasses which are supposed to help you see auras." She handed me the glasses to put on, then posed expectantly at the required distance away from me so that I could see her aura. I didn't see a thing! Her hopes were dashed. In a way, mine were too.

Nothing Adelle did ever surprised me. Secretly, she was always seeking to be a more spiritual person. Once when her husband was driving us along a razorback mountain road, with sheer cliffs dropping precipitously on both sides below us, and no place to turn around to get back to safety, Adelle became terrified, and said, "Linda, tell me everything you know about prayer!"

Occasionally, only, have I seen an aura, then very faint, and emanating only from highly powered individuals such as spiritual teachers or ministers. But I still longed to see them readily and easily and fully. What I am going to tell you now has never been made public before. I am sharing with you these experiences only to assure you that if something unusual happens to you, as it is happening to so many these days, there is no need to panic. Even if you hope for or expect it, it never seems to happen as you expect.

Not too long ago, I had my turn. Healing is my number one interest whether it is nutritional, spiritual or via color. While I was doing research on color therapy for my color book, I was interviewing people who had long been working in this field. Disappointingly, I was not allowed to mention them due to the rigid rules enforced by the medical monopoly, which I have explained in that book. However, one of these practitioners, who is highly successful, came to my hotel room while I was in her city and explained her method of color healing to me. After we were through, we went to the hotel dining room for dinner. The room was illuminated by candles only, one at each table. As I faced this woman who was talking, I suddenly said, "I am sorry, but I haven't heard a word you said for the last ten minutes." She looked alarmed and asked why.

I said, "At first I thought it was due to the flickering candles, but now I am sure it is not. I see intense color radiating from your hands and fingers and I have never seen anything like it before."

She laughed and said, "Oh, that's because I work so much with color for healing." She asked what the color was and I explained that it was a flame color. She didn't seem surprised. I was the one who was surprised!

Not long afterward, I stopped at a friend's house in my own community to return a borrowed book. The friend, a highly spiritual person and physical therapist with some healing ability of her own, came to the door, accepted the book with one hand, and in that hand (not the other) I saw the same color—a flame red, emanating from her hand too! I left in a somewhat shaken state. Imagination? No.

The next instance occurred when a doctor (an M.D. who uses natural methods only, no drugs, no surgery) and his wife were at my house for lunch. We were all standing in the kitchen talking when suddenly I saw the same color coming from both of his hands. I did not tell him because I knew he would not have believed it. A few minutes later, I happened to catch sight of my own hands, and I saw the same color there! How I got through the meal, I am not sure. I was shaking like a leaf.

Since then, the experience has become routine. Yet, if I look for colors I never see them. They only appear when unexpectedly I see them out of the corner of my eye, so I don't try to see them. If I look straight at the hands, no colors. And I do not see color in everyone. Since I am privileged to entertain some special people, I am a bit fussy about whom I invite to my house. People who are curiosity seekers, negative thinkers, or sappers (those who sap energy from anyone they can to shore up their own) I leave strictly alone. My work allows little time for entertaining, anyway, and I see no one without appointment or for a very good reason. I mention this, since the number of colors radiating from hands, which I have witnessed in my own living room is remarkably high. Not only are these people special, as a rule, but they are usually highly spiritual as well.

One friend, a clairvoyant healer and a minister, radiates different colors at different times. Each time she comes, it is a different color. Another clairvoyant, internationally known and one who does occasional healing, alternates between two colors only. At one visit she radiates a golden color from her hands and lower arms; at another it will be a soft lavender. I do not know why.

A man, who for years exhibited no color at all that I could see, experienced a spiritual awakening when he was praying for someone else who was healed as a result. He had also been suffering from a mystifying disturbance himself for several years, which no one could diagnose or relieve. He, too, was healed of this ailment, not because he was praying for himself, but for the other person who was in serious danger following a heart attack. So both were healed to the amazement of attending doctors.

It was not long afterward that this man came to my house, and for the first time since I had known him (about ten years) golden color poured out of his hands and arms. My white Siamese cat wandered in about that time and jumped up on his lap. He held the cat for about half an hour, and so help me, when the cat jumped to the floor, it, too, had absorbed the color and turned golden! Later, the cat returned. The gold color had disappeared and has never returned.

When Yvonne came to visit, she was talking rapidly about one condition after another, and the colors in her hands changed just as rapidly, like a kaleidoscope.

As I recall, the colors jumped from turquoise, to green, to lavender, and others. I tried to keep up with them, calling them out as they appeared. Fortunately, she was not impatient at being interrupted every few words, since I was reporting excitedly something I had not witnessed before.

I am sure my experiences are not unique, but they were years in coming. I am truly grateful for them and the message they convey to me, when the color shines from a person's hand is: "This person is a healer." But, one does not have to know if his hands radiate color, in order to heal. Blessing someone, mentally, or audibly; or helping them with a problem; or soothing their distress; even praying for them to remove their fear or worry, all of these things are forms of healing and anyone can do it!

9.

finding
YOUR WAY

Today, as we now know, many people are opening up spiritually. Yet no two open up in the same way, at the same rate of speed. Some of us have taken almost a lifetime to learn how to be more spiritual, which often includes a heightened intuition, seeing auras, feeling a sense of guidance and other experiences, new to us. One woman, working with color to help elderly people lose their fear of death, did not "open up" until she was fifty. She suddenly began seeing and conversing with angels, who guided her in her new career in color to which she has dedicated herself unselfishly. Yet she states that many young people have now been born already armed with such knowledge. Those who believe in reincarnation believe that they have earned the knowledge in another life and have brought it with them.

There is a vast difference between spiritual growth and psychic experience. Spiritual growth is on the highest possible, safest level. Psychic development, even black magic, is on a much lower level, sometimes possibly leading into danger. Spiritual development does not come easily. One has to earn it, and it often appears only after prolonged suffering of one type or another, as if it were a test before one is worthy of initiation into the wonders of the Divine Hierarchy. Once on the "Spiritual path," as it is called, the way is rocky, but the rewards which come later, are great, according to those who have been through it. The adepts state that you are tested and tested until you are convinced you can stand no more suffering, yet no one is given a test beyond his endurance. It is a means of separating the wheat from the chaff, the men from the boys.

There are many books which hint at such spiritual experiences and growth, but none which actually chart your exact course for you, because each person develops differently from another and from the *inside out*, not the outside inward. Some unseen helper or force seems to be guiding you and knows you better than you know yourself.

As you go along, you realize more and more that you are not alone. If you pray for guidance and protection and turn your life over to a higher power "according to the will of the Father" or "in Jesus Christ's name" or whatever is meaningful in your religious belief, you will not be disappointed as long as you don't get in your own light and insist on doing things *your* way. It is necessary to maintain a "not my will but Thine be done" attitude.

.People will come to you at the right time to fill a need in your life, although never as you expect. A book which has information you need at any particular stage of your growth will almost jump off a bookshelf at you, or as you turn the pages of a book you already have (the Bible in particular) a message will seem to jump off the page to catch your attention. On a more mundane level, you may forget your car keys, and grumblingly return to the house to get them perhaps only to learn later that by that short delay you avoided a traffic accident.

Don't take our word for this; ask anyone whom you suspect is "on the path" and is interested in spiritual subjects; they will confirm it.

Once I was in a bookshop looking for a paperback copy of an ESP book. I had read a borrowed copy in hardback but now wanted a paperback edition for my library. I looked on the shelf where such books were kept in the bookstore, but the shelf was empty. As I inquired at the counter if they had a copy elsewhere, a middle-aged man standing next to me held out a copy toward me. He said "I took the last copy. You may have it."

I thanked him but said "Oh, no, you found it first, *You* take it. I will wait for another shipment."

He answered, "Oh, no, *you* take it!" We continued this Gaston-and-Alphonse routine for a while, until he said, "Look, you might as well take it. *I don't find books; they find me.*"

I finally consented. After he walked out I asked the

clerk at the counter who the man was; his philosophy seemed so different from that of the usual person.

The clerk said, "I don't know his name, but he is a retired priest."

Another example of this speed-up in momentum of spiritual growth is the fact that spiritual healers are popping up everywhere. Book after book is being published telling how some have been working at it for years, while others seem to have suddenly acquired the healing ability in a few short months. Many are having fantastic results, and no one is more surprised that the healer himself. The fact that the ability came out of the blue without much warning is almost too much to believe. But these healers are developing at the right time. Everyone seems to be sick these days.

Most spiritual healers have to operate underground since the medical monopoly will not brook interference with their surgical and drug treatments and are ready to persecute anyone who represents competition. Yet, properly used, there should be room for both types of healing. Some doctors are actually calling upon spiritual healers for diagnosis before performing unnecessary surgery or "surgical exploration," in order to find the cause of an elusive ailment. In a few cases, other doctors are sending patients whom they cannot help to healers. Even more surprising, some doctors themselves are demonstrating spiritual healing ability, but dare not admit it for fear of retribution from "the establishment." The time may come, in fact it is already beginning, when patients will prefer doctors who use such healing techniques. People are already flocking to spiritual healers to avoid unnecessary surgery, dangerous drugs, and painful, expensive and inadequate medical tests.

I have told the story elsewhere about the client of a spiritually evolved counselor, now deceased, who promised to pray for her client who was to undergo brain surgery. The client was understandably frightened because of the operation, and the counselor consoled him by promising to also pray for his physician so that he would be spiritually guided to perform the operation successfully.

Several days after the operation (which was successful) the surgeon came to the patient's hospital room. He seemed greatly agitated. He asked his patient, "Can you give me any explanation of what occurred during your operation?"

The man answered in surprise, "I don't know what you are talking about."

The surgeon said, "When I started using my scalpel, a white light flashed from it and remained there until the operation was finished. I have never before had such an experience in my entire career."

The patient laughed, "Oh," he said, "that was the result of a prayer by my spiritual counselor who promised to help us both during the operation."

The doctor was so stunned that he asked for the name of the counselor, later visited her, and asked her to guide him to a more spiritual life. She started him off with the Bible.

There are many forms of healing. Color therapy is one form, but it is banned in this country by the medical monopoly. Professionals dare not use it to treat others, so this book does not provide information on how to treat others with color. However, who is to know if you are treating yourself and breathing color? As mentioned earlier, others can stop us from using color equipment, but no one can stop us from breathing!

The most successful methods of healing are spiritual, not by personal magnetism. Personal magnetic healing is that which employs the healer's own energy or magnetism, leaving the healer exhausted after the treatment and usually producing only a temporary healing in the patient. Spiritual healing, on the other hand, tunes into a higher power, usually of Divine source, and is requested by, and channeled through the healer to the patient. This higher power has different names such as prana (taken from the yoga) or Life Force, or Universal Life Energy, or Divine Power emanating from God. The terminology is chosen by those who use it according to their own beliefs, yet it may be one and the same substance. The healing breath we have discussed in previous chapters can also be classified under one of these categories.

To our knowledge, however, *no healing with color breathing has proved successful unless the person also combines color with spiritual know-how,* as explained throughout this book. One explanation: the late Eleanore Thedick, a clairvoyant and color expert, wrote that there are bands of angels, called the Color Angels, who are assigned to work with colors exclusively. These angels, she believed, are also constantly beaming vitalizing color toward the earth during these trying times when fear, pessimism and other negative conditions are rampant.

Another possible explanation; a healer friend described the simple secret of healing as follows: it is merely based upon raising the vibration of a cell, organ or gland which is ailing due to a lowered vibration caused by shock, injury, malnutrition, negative thought or many other reasons. Since color is a source of vibration, it is not surprising that it can either raise the vibration when necessary, or neutralize a disturbing vibration, and thus become a factor in healing. But, if it is coupled with another form of higher energy also high in vibration, results may be dramatic. This is why, when most color healers are at work, they not only visualize the result as perfect and being successfully accomplished but add such statements as "this is now healed according to the will of the Father," or "in His name" or in "Jesus Christ's Name," one of the highest vibrations ever known. In this way you are not taking the responsibility for the healing yourself, but turning it over to a higher power, where it belongs. After all, we should not play God since we do not know everything there is to know about our own body or anyone else's. "It is God who doeth the works."

There is no doubt that color already is classified as an art, but it may be rapidly becoming a science. Perhaps, as stated in *Color Therapy*, as a science, it will be a revival of that practiced many centuries ago. Perhaps it will even reach new heights. It is too soon to tell.

Let us add a solemn warning. Color has vibration, as you now know. Thought also has vibration. If you send a color or a thought accompanied with a wish for evil to another person, it will be returned to you with accrued interest. The boomerang, even if sent to another, will occur to *you*, perhaps promptly or with delayed action, but the law is immutable; it will return to the sender! So use the laws of vibration for the good of others as well as yourself. If you sow good, you will receive it. If you sow evil or negativity, even for yourself, you will also receive that. You are the computer.

The fact that you are reading this book is a hopeful sign. It means that undoubtedly you are interested in color. But you are no doubt also interested in getting results with the use of color breathing. To assure success, let us suggest that you use this art, or new science, not for personal reasons only, but to become a better person and to help mankind as well. Hitch your wagon to a star, combine color breathing with the use of a higher spiritual power, and join the growing throng which is trying to help the world become a better place in which to live.

We send you our love, our blessings and our wishes for success.

Linda and Yvonne

Note: Unfortunately, due to crowded schedules we cannot correspond with readers. If, however, you wish to share with us your discoveries in color breathing which were helpful for you, we would be glad to see them. Please address us in care of the publisher.

NOTES

1. Linda Clark, *Color Therapy* (Old Greenwich, Connecticut: Devin Adair, Co., 1974).
2. Linda Clark, *Help Yourself to Health* (New York: Pyramid Pubns. 1974).
3. Roland Hunt, *Man Made Clear for the Nu-Clear Age* (Lakemont, Georgia: CSA Press, 1969).
4. Jess Stearn, *Yoga, Youth and Reincarnation* (New York: Doubleday & Company, Inc., 1965).
5. Linda Clark, *Secrets of Health & Beauty* (New York: Pyramid Pubns. 1970).
6. Linda Clark and Kay Lee, *Beauty Questions and Answers* (New York: Pyramid Pubns.).
7 Hans Holzer, *The Human Dynamo* (Millbrae, California: Celestial Arts, 1975).
8 Linda Clark, *Get Well Naturally*, (New York: Arc Books, 1968).

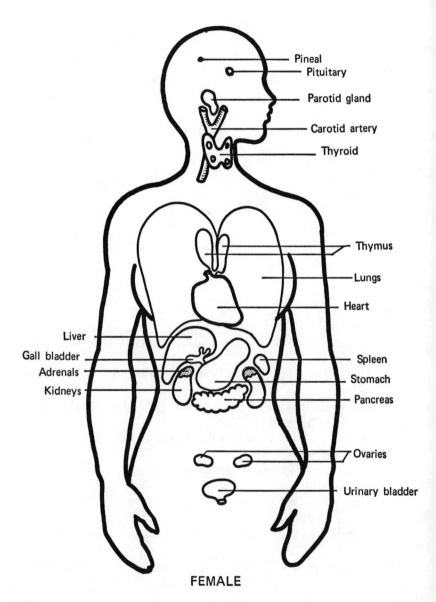

Pineal
Pituitary
Parotid gland
Carotid artery
Thyroid
Thymus
Lungs
Heart
Liver
Gall bladder
Adrenals
Kidneys
Spleen
Stomach
Pancreas
Ovaries
Urinary bladder

FEMALE

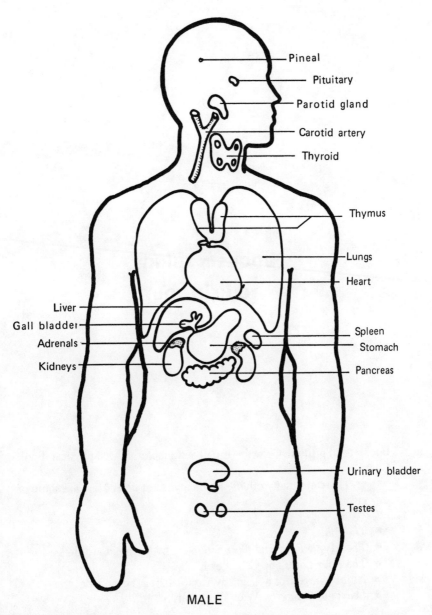

MALE

books 'n things
to help you

Books for Spiritual Growth (usually available at Metaphysical Book Shops)

There are many others, too many to list here. Here are some of our favorites:

- *The Bible.*
- *The Mystic Path and Cosmic Power,* by Verne Howard
- *The Four Loves,* by C.S. Lewis
- *Autobiography* of a Yogi, by Paramahansa Yogananda
- *Leaves of Grass,* by Walt Whitman

- *Cosmic Consciousness*, by Richard Bucke
- *Wisdom of the Mystic Masters*, (paperback edition) Joseph J. Weed.
  —A fascinating book based on the teachings of the Rosicrucians

- *Let's Eat Right to Keep Fit*, by Adelle Davis.
- *The Human Dynamo*, by Hans Holzer, Ph.D. (Paperback)
  —Deals with spiritual power and how to get what you want.
- *Help Yourself to Health*, by Linda Clark
  —An ESP book including chapter on angels. (Paperback)
- *Watch Your Dreams*, by Ann Ree Colton
  —Explaining dreams and their symbols.
- *Ethical ESP*, by Ann Ree Colton
  —The difference between lower and higher ESP.
- *The Human Spirit*, by Ann Ree Colton
  —A scientific, spiritual and healing book on the creation, purpose and destiny of man.
- *The Jesus Story*, by Ann Ree Colton
  (All Ann Ree Colton's books may be ordered from *Niscience*, 336 W. Colorado St., Glendale, Calif. 91204. Write for prices.)

- *The Seven Keys to Color*, by Roland T. Hunt.
- *The Eighth Key to Color*, by Roland T. Hunt

Records

1. A complete course via cassette tapes on Color from a reliable source: Christ Ministry Foundation, P.O. Box 1103, Santa Cruz, California, 95061.

Name of Course:		"THE REALITY OF COLOR"	Price
Tape 1	Side 1	"Color as Light—Light as God"	$4.65
	2	Meditation, "The Power of the Rays"	
2	Side 1	"Color and the Aura"	4.65
	2	Meditation, "Waves of Color"	
3	Side 1	"Our Seven Auras"	4.65
	2	Meditation, "Healing Our Auras"	

4	Side 1	"Meaning of the Seven Color Rays"	4.65
	2	Meditation, "A Trip to a Temple of Color"	
5	Side 1	"Techniques of Color Healing"	4.65
	2	Meditation, "The Breathing of Colors"	
6	Side 1	"Color, Music, Numbers, the Zodiac"	4.65
	2	"Relaxation and Color"	
7	Side 1	"The Reality of Spiritual Broadcasting"	4.65
	2	"We Send out Color as Service"	

Price, $4.65 each tape, postpaid. Tax $.26 each tape for California residents. Entire set $26.00, tax $1.56 for California residents.

2. *"Christening for Listening: A Sound track for Every Body"*
A LP record of short compositions keyed to each of the soul colors, and attuned to the corresponding musical scale note. Composed by psychologist-musician Steven Halpern. This record has been used in its entirety by psychiatrist , and plant nurseries to encourage plant growth. It has soothed ravelled nerves, served as a natural tranquilizer to some, even stopping babies from crying. Also considered helpful for meditation. Unique. Available from Open Channel Sound Co., 1625 Middlefield Rd., Palo Alto, Calif., 94301 $5.00 postpaid.

The Pendulum

1. A recent book: *Psychologistics*, An Operating Manual for the Mind, by T.A. Waters. Available from Random House, 201 East 50th Street, N.Y., N.Y. 10022. Hardback. $7.95.
2. *Get Well Naturally*, by Linda Clark. Paperback edition. See chapter on pendulum entitled, "Do It Yourself Radiesthesia."

3. To buy a pendulum: a beautiful "tear drop" well balanced plastic pendulum, mailed in a red velvet box. A lifetime possession. Order from HR Enterprises, Inc., Box 4321, Fullerton, California 92634. Price $7.95 postpaid.

INDEX